Four Gates to Health

Eastern Ideas and Techniques for Vital Living

Four Gates to Health

Eastern Ideas and Techniques for Vital Living

Julian Lynn

Nymphaea Works

Springfield, Missouri

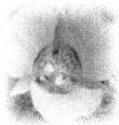

Author: Julian Lynn
Photographer: Julian Lynn

Cataloging-in-Publication Data
Lynn, Julian
    Four gates to health: eastern ideas and techniques for
vital living. / Julian Lynn. -1st ed.

ISBN 978-0-578-12097-3

1. Self-care, Health. 2. Breathing exercises.
I. Lynn, Julian. II. Title.

2011912917

Dewey-Decimal-System Classification: 613

questions@julianlynn.com
orders@nymphaeaworks.com
© 2013, Julian Lynn

ISBN: 978-0-578-12097-3

Dedication

To all of my students—
you have served consistently as my most
generous, invaluable and patient teachers.

Table of Contents

Introduction

During the last summer of my teaching college-level yoga, I noticed my students growing and changing in ways which could not be explained by the practice of yoga's physical postures alone. This change was something I had observed over the course of many semesters, but only after enjoying a particularly successful, intensive summer class did I then acknowledge the relationship between class attendance and the visible changes in my students' faces. Reflective awareness was taking the place of preoccupation. Around the edges of class, students talked openly about positive changes in their lives which they attributed to the successful application of ideas and techniques presented in class. Everyone had a glow about them. Despite the fact that most students were carrying full course loads, everyone was becoming more radiant.

Each class has its own personality. With the yoga classes I taught, students were able to enroll again and again. For some classes, especially those heavily populated with returning students, the regular practice of yoga's physical postures is enough to pull an evolved and engaged group of souls back to center. The most advanced "swimmers" among them carry the beginning students into the calm, deep end of the still, meditative pool. This is one of the things that the practice of yoga is capable of doing.

As an instructor, I had already developed a profound faith in the practice of yoga and the power of Vedic tradition's many and varied breathing techniques to transform lives. I had also come to respect my students as my most patient teachers. They listened to lectures that fell flat, showed me what real discipline can do and taught me to persevere on days when I was far from center. During that last summer class, we met almost daily, and I was finally able to make the correlation between regular class attendance and the most marked, radiant facial expressions among my most frequent students.

At a semester's close, it is not unusual to hear a student remark, "Thank you for the life lessons. They were helpful." or "I really liked some of the ideas that were covered in class." These comments are also part of formal academic review. On several occasions, I received requests for "the book" or "a book" that would aid with the review of ideas discussed in class. Truth be known, there is no single book, but there have been many books, articles, seminars and contemplative experiences over the years. The majority of these I read, reviewed, attended and had years prior to becoming a yoga instructor.

As a reader, it may be helpful for you to know that I personally read in the areas of Eastern philosophy, general biography, cultural studies, anthropology and, what some would term, esoteric studies. I also enjoy a good article in a "muscle" magazine. What interests me is how individual cultures and people relate to their experiences as they move through life's passages.

A trial by fire caused me to embark on additional reading in the areas of wellness, nutrition, traditional Chinese medicine and alternative healthcare. Subsequent to all of this reading, I had a series of singular contemplative experiences which caused me to begin attending seminars in a variety of Eastern philosophical traditions. I was on a quest to find accurately descriptive vocabulary and documentation of others' parallel contemplative experiences.

This compilation provides a selection of ideas and breathing techniques which my own students found transformational. The format is designed as an aid to individuals who are beginning or already enjoying an established fitness program but who may not have the luxury of time or means to attend seminars and review stacks of literature. With the possible exception of the concept of the Four Gates, most of the material in this book is well documented in a variety of sources on Eastern philosophical theory and within the realm of popular psychology. To the purists in each of these traditions and fields, I offer an apology for the fusing of approaches and departure from traditional vocabulary. The few notes I chose to include on aspects of Vedic theory are there as points of interest and contrast. Read these notes with an open mind and the same intellectual curiosity that you would bring to a book on anthropology.

That being said, it is because of the many words and acts of encouragement from my students that I decided to formalize a selection of my lecture notes. In the end, it was the chance meetings with various students from semesters long past that made the difference—whether it was a graceful bow at the dog park with a confession about how much someone missed my classes "because no one teaches yoga quite like you" or an unexpected and respectful hug on a public street. Such expressions of appreciation come as a result of students' having connected with their own immutable purity—their own sweetness. This is a gift that I wish everyone could have and hold—an experience of essence. I am hopeful that the offerings in this volume will draw you closer to your Self.

If you are able, read the ideas and attempt the techniques in the order presented. Think of the relationship between them as the parallel tracks for a single train. Sequencing is important. I am hopeful that the book will act as a springboard to the wealth of literature, opportunities and practices in the traditions and fields mentioned. To that end, I have included a brief Recommended Miscellany.

Remember to support yourself with kind words and buoy yourself up, on the worst of days, with your own fierceness and tenacity. Please use only the ideas and techniques that you deem appropriate and release the rest.

Julian Lynn
March 2012

Toward an Integrated Self

Incredible things happen whenever we commit to a fitness routine or an ongoing exercise program. Most of us approach the fitness studio or health center thinking we are simply working on physical issues, such as maintaining bone density, improving flexibility, trimming off a few pounds or improving muscle tone. Then, one day, in the middle of our solo run on the elliptical machine or on the mat during a group fitness class, we find ourselves experiencing a greater joy than we have ever known or an unnamed sorrow that is baffling—origins unknown.

Whether or not we anticipate it, strengthening the physical body causes us to begin the process of shedding experiential and emotional shadows that were once sequestered away in the body's fabric—or tissues. During the strengthening process, our bodies actually begin to create space for new experiences and our individual essence. As a result of our dedication to our physical routine, forgotten moments of intense emotional range are presented to be reorganized and compressed into files of a smaller and more impersonal type. For some, old memories may push forward and require resolution. For others, a quiet review of behavior becomes part of our mental routine during a workout, fostering greater responsibility and thoughtfulness in our actions and manners than we previously employed or thought possible. Whatever our experience may be, joy begins to express itself in an ever-intensifying and more frequent manner as we make a shift, seating the essence into the body. And, when joy becomes the predominant emotional experience during the course of everyday living, we know we have come to center. With this shift, we experience a feeling of wholeness—an integrated sense of Self.

Different traditions have their own descriptions and vocabularies for this process of unfolding or transformation which includes the migration of the essence into the body. In Vedic tradition, the physical postures of yoga are practiced to strengthen the body, so we can sit in meditation and prepare to hold the higher Self or Atman. In Sufism, an aspirant looks to establish a connection with the Essential Self and release the false idol of the ego or Commanding Self. In Christian terms, one of the best parallel understandings appears in Quaker tradition (Religious Society of Friends), where the essence is referred to as The Light of Christ. Like Vedic theory, Quaker tradition holds the understanding that this Light is present in each of us.

Whatever vocabulary we choose to describe this process of becoming integrated is of a secondary concern. What matters is that we have made the commitment to embark on a voyage of self-discovery. As a result of our commitment to strengthening the body, we will most likely encounter the Self and begin asking the twin questions: Who am I? And, why am I here? Our answers to these fundamental questions hinge upon our ability to connect directly with the body and the breath.

With the best of variables in place, such as support and personal discipline, pursuit of a dedicated fitness program may be life-changing. In connecting with our own life force, we are preparing to experience, potentially, one note-worthy moment after another. The pacing of breakthrough moments varies. Sometimes they come in rapid succession like a cascade, followed by seemingly long phases of dry division. The ideas and techniques in this book are designed to smooth the pacing and ease the transitions during your process of transformation.

We know when we have had an experience of wholeness or integrated Self by relying on the descriptions furnished by other students of body and breath work who have gone before us. Some students of this integrative process describe the experience as one of profound calmness or quiet stillness. Others describe this feeling as being in "the zone" or a place where there is no sense of time. Becoming fully centered and grounded causes us to realize our own strength or "power." This is not a strength that needs exertion over anything or anyone else, but a feeling of solidness within one's Self. Some, especially those who have not been allowed to express the volition of their essence, may experience some anger when the Self is first uncovered.

From a physical point of view, the most important thing that happens with the invitation of the essence into the body is that we begin making decisions that are consistent with the affirmation of our own vitality and, from a

5

psychological point of view, our behavior begins to affirm our uniqueness—without our feeling the need to orchestrate, control or interfere with anyone else. For example, we may begin making dietary and lifestyle choices based upon the body's very specific need at a given point in time, as well as working to release habituated patterns of behavior and relationship.

As time lapses and our physical body gains strength, we change our previously automatic agreement to or engagement in less-than-optimal habits and lifestyle patterns. Having developed a heightened sense of body awareness, old habits are replaced by new ones—whether in personal or interpersonal behavior. Anger dissipates. Grief is released. Joy unfolds. We develop internal steadiness. We actively begin to make thoughtful choices about the what, where, when and who in our lives. We may even choose to set a distinctly altered life course.

Breathing into the Belly: This breathing technique invites us into the body and helps build self-awareness regarding our abdominal muscles and breathing rhythms. Practiced in a fully reclining position, this exercise is extraordinary in its efficacy. If you are new to your physical routine, you will learn to recognize and feel your postural muscles in action. In a limited and gentle way, belly breathing also helps us become aware of the muscles serving the lower belly. If your core strength is less than optimal, it is advisable to find a safe method for strengthening your abdominal muscles. Some of the seated exercises later in the book are best enjoyed with these postural muscles already developed. Be sure to have a light, mid-sized textbook, small bean bag, stuffed lap desk or another book to use as a prop.

Caution: If you have preexisting abdominal concerns, conditions or injuries, do not use any type of prop on your lower belly and consult with a physician before attempting this exercise.

Toward an Integrated Self

- Find a suitable location, where you may recline comfortably for approximately seven to twelve minutes. Before practicing, begin by clearing your nose thoroughly.

- If you need to support your head with a thin pillow, you may. Otherwise, enjoy this exercise with your body laid flat. Your spine is straight and long. Your toes fall away from the center or midline of your body.

- Place the light textbook, bean bag, lap desk or telephone book on your belly, below your navel. Inhaling through your nose, imagine bringing your breath all of the way down to the top of your pubic bone and observe the prop rising with your inhalation. As you exhale, observe your chosen prop falling. The breath is steady and even.

- Allow the length of the exhalation to match your inhalation. Adjust or change the prop you have selected until you find one that feels like a good fit for your body. There should be no strain on the inhaling breath and a comfortable sense of gentle resistance when exhaling evenly.

▪ Observe each time as you inhale. The abdomen and ribs are expanding. With each exhale, your belly and chest are contracting. Continue inhaling and exhaling for five to seven minutes without pausing between breaths. If you are normally a shallow breather, reduce the time to three to five minutes and exercise caution when first trying this technique.

▪ When you have completed this exercise, remove the prop and carefully roll to your right or left side, whichever is most comfortable. Pause here to take two or three additional cycles of breath. (A cycle of breath consists of one exhale and one inhale.)

▪ Using your arms, come to a seated position. Remain seated and take three to seven additional cycles of breath to ensure that you are fully aware of your surroundings and grounded in your body.

▪ As you work with this exercise, you may expand the length of time that you spend breathing with the same prop on your abdomen. Expand your practice time, working between twelve and fifteen minutes.

Toward an Integrated Self

Then, try practicing up to a total of twenty-one minutes. (Do not increase the weight of the prop. The prop is there as a tool to build breath and core awareness, not to increase muscle strength.)

Approaching the Four Gates

Good or bad. Right or wrong. If we have grown up immersed in American popular culture or have even lived adjacent to it, we know how deeply engrained this manner of dualistic thinking can become and how difficult it may be to change.

Early in our childhoods, the conceptual dualism of good and bad is one of the first frameworks for thinking that we encounter. Our early behavior is labeled using this system of categorization. We choose sides and play games through the prism of this concept. The concept of duality also appears consistently in children's media. At its best, the dualistic framework acts as a simple sorting tool so that we, as children, may choose socially appropriate thoughts to entertain, words to say, actions to take and individuals to befriend. When this method of thinking still occupies an active place in our adult minds, it may contribute to our being overly simplistic in how we approach problem solving. At its worst, dualistic thinking may contribute to our becoming judgmental toward ourselves or others.

For young children, the concept serves as a simplified method for sorting through early experiences. There is no ill intent on the part of our guardians or society in teaching us this shorthand. Most of our childhood caregivers are working with the genuine intent of helping us make our way in a complex world.

In addition to being part of our cultural tradition, dualism is also a deep-seated part of our linguistic tradition, accompanied by the pairing of right and wrong. My first revelation regarding right and wrong occurred while studying another language. After learning how to say good and bad, I was anticipating learning how to say right and wrong. Amazingly, in this non-Germanic linguistic tradition, there was no discrete word for "wrong." A person may do something the right way or not the right way. Linguistically and theoretically, there is more room in that language for variation in behavior and outcome than is implied in English.

Our birth language or primary first language shapes the ways in which we construct and perceive our world, as well as influencing how we behave or relate to the world. While it is true that, at the time of my study, right and wrong did not exist as a linguistic pairing in this language, there were other linguistic precepts and grammatical structures holding this linguistic culture in check. Most notably there was a strong adherence to tradition, lack of grammatical acceptance for personal responsibility—as evidenced by the pervasive use of passive sentence structures—and a genuine fear of standing out. Two aphorisms come to mind from this culture. One involves reminding children that "I" is the last letter in the (their) alphabet and, another, warning that the tall nail receives the blow.

Over the course of a hectic day, most of our decisions are made in rapid succession based upon habituated patterns of thought, belief and behavior which we may not have reexamined in a very long time. When we are operating on autopilot, we rely on the would-be preassembled judicial scales in our heads to make decisions for us rather than actually living in our bodies and taking the time to make reflective choices based on a given situation. When we are not fully grounded in the body, we further compromise ourselves by abdicating our body's authority to predetermined cultural and personal behavioral patterns, as well as relying on dualistic thinking. Thus, we are often unable to make decisions that are optimal for us at a given time—decisions that have the potential to foster enhanced vitality.

Is it good or bad? Is it right or wrong? If our decision-making process is more uniquely nuanced than most, we personalize the good-bad framework by adding the phrases "for me" or "at this time." In this way, the decisions we make are given a greater degree of thought with reference to our specific circumstances. For the purposes of this chapter's discussion, consider replacing a dualistic approach to problem solving with the system of the Four Gates.

Before reading about the system of the Four Gates ask yourself the following questions: What energizes me? What makes me radiant and joyful? And, what fills me with life? Begin thinking in terms of enhancing your personal vitality or life force—because embracing your own vibrancy brings you closer to yourself at the level of essence.

In order to foster thinking skills which, rely upon what is appropriate for us at a given time, we must work on the assumption that we want to do what is inherently best for ourselves, our bodies and life force. The system of the Four Gates is designed to be used in day-to-day living, replacing dualistic thinking and preconditioned choice patterns. Work through this list of questions the next time you are making a decision in the grocery store or thinking about participating in a defined activity or joining a group venture.

- What is the short-term effect on my vitality if I ...?
- What is the long-term effect on my vitality if I ...?
- What is the short-term effect on society's vitality if I ...?
- What is the long-term effect on society's vitality if I ...?

These are the Four Gates that our personal decisions should pass through. Initially, taking time to go through the list may feel cumbersome. Adherence to working through these questions helps move us into our physical bodies, further grounding us, so that even seemingly small decisions may be followed by a boost in personal vitality. The reference to society or community places our personal decisions into a context. The reference to short-term and long-term vitality gives us a sense of the trajectory for our decisions' results through time.

At this point, let's work through a scenario. The scenario is purposefully direct so that it is easy to see the logic behind the application of the system of the Four Gates. If the scenario is outside of the realm of your experience, you may create an example of your own design and apply the questions as you progress through it.

Imagine that you have spent an entire afternoon working in the garden under the hot sun. Some friends stop by your house at five, asking you out for half-price tap beer at a local cantina and eatery. You offer to meet them in one-half hour. After a shower, you change clothes and drive to your meeting place. Soon, you are enjoying complimentary hors d'oeuvres and half-price beer under a beautiful sky at their street-side café. Remember, you are hot, tired and very hungry from all of the yard work.

As time lapses, one glass of beer turns into four glasses (or it could be wine)—inside of one hour.   Although you have been snacking, the alcohol enters your system more quickly than the nutrients from the food. While quenching your thirst and feeding your body, you have forgotten all about using the system of the Four Gates.

For discussion purposes, let's work through the questions in the system of the Four Gates after the fact. What is the short-term effect on your vitality of what you have consumed? Your body is working hard to metabolize everything that you have eaten and drunk. The excessive alcohol consumption has compromised your body. Assuming you routinely follow a balanced diet, live in a clean environment and enjoy a few days that are alcohol free, you will likely recover. What is the long-term effect on your vitality of the last hour's drinking and eating? If "happy hour" is not a regular part of your lifestyle, this singular outing should not have an adverse effect on your long-term vitality, given factors such as a normally healthy diet and environment.

Next, you get up from the table and begin to feel the alcohol in your system. What is the short-term effect on society's vitality? There are several possible answers or outcomes. As you weave down the street, you could prove to be an embarrassment to your friends—especially if you were to become sick on the street curb. Or, your friends may feel inconvenienced in the event that you require a ride home. If you require a taxi ride home, the literal cost of your behavior goes up with the addition of taxi expenses.

Let's change the scenario and consider the last question in the system of the Four Gates. What is the long-term effect on society's vitality if you choose to drive home? You can see where this decision might lead. Remember, you are intoxicated and your judgment is seriously impaired. If you choose to drive home and there is an accident, this single action could have life-altering consequences, not only for you, but for the lives of many people—if there are fatalities.

This is an overstated example, but it is a valuable one. Even seemingly minor decisions—those made while standing in front of a vending machine at three-thirty in the afternoon—become potentially life changing. When we consistently opt for the sweet delight cakes filled with artificially-flavored cream for an afternoon snack, we must consider the ramifications of our behaviors in the big picture. What happens if one seemingly small daily or twice-weekly habit contributes to our becoming diabetic? Begin thinking things through in terms of personal vitality and long-term impact. And, maybe the next time the afternoon munchies hit and the vending machine calls, you may find yourself choosing packaged nuts. Or, you may even opt to pack a vitality-boosting snack from home for each day's afternoon break.

Understand the implications of seemingly small choices. Use the system of the Four Gates to begin assessing your patterns of behavior and long-standing habits. With measured and consistent application, the questions can assist you in making better personal choices with greater confidence. Committing to a shift in thinking, so that personal vitality becomes primary, is about embracing the full potential of your life force. By embracing your own life force, you will gain the energetic reserves you need to benefit your essence and honor the care and deep concern of those around you, who also support your long-term health and well-being.

Breathing into the Body: This breathing technique brings us into the body in an unhurried and invitational manner. It is practiced in a fully reclining position. If you are still new to your fitness program, this exercise does not require the postural muscles that some of the later breathing techniques do.

- Find a suitable location, where you may recline comfortably for approximately twelve to fifteen minutes. Have tissue at hand, so that you may clear your nose thoroughly before beginning.

Approaching the Four Gates

- If you need to support your head with a thin pillow, you may do so. Otherwise, enjoy this practice with your body laid out completely flat. Be sure that your body and spine are straight and long. Allow your toes to fall away from the midline of your body.

- Place the palms of your hands on your lower belly with the fingers gently spread. The tips of your middle fingers may touch or your fingers may interlace. Exhale to clear your lungs. On an inhaling breath, allow your lower belly to inflate. Think about bringing the breath all the way down to your pubic bone. The inhalation is thorough, steady and even. Your lungs are comfortably full.

- On your exhaling breath, allow the length of the exhalation to match that of your inhalation. Gently contract your abdominal muscles to wash the air up and out of the tops of your lungs. Your hands should fall naturally when you contract your abdominal muscles on the exhalation.

- Breathe in this manner for three full minutes without pausing between breaths.

- After three minutes, gently slide your hands above your navel, at the base of the ribs. Shift your focus, bringing your breath into the middle body. Observe that each time, as you inhale, your hands are rising and the ribs are expanding. With each exhale, the hands are falling and the ribs are contracting.

- Now, continue breathing smoothly and evenly into your middle body for an additional three minutes.

- Next, place your hands on the area of the chest below your collar bones. On your inhalation, focus on bringing the breath into the upper lungs to the area under your hands. With each exhalation, your hands should fall. Continue concentrating your breath and attention in this region of the torso for three minutes.

- When you have completed this final phase of the breathing practice, roll carefully to your right or left side, whichever is more comfortable. Pause to take two to three cycles of breath on your side; and then, using your arms, come to a seated position.

• Take an additional three to seven cycles of breath, while seated, to ensure that you are fully grounded in your body and aware of your surroundings.

• As you work with this exercise, you may expand the length of time that you spend in each area of the torso to the duration most appropriate for your body (approximately five to seven minutes per area).

Note: As a result of our acculturation, many of us attempt to align ourselves with our perception of "goodness" so that we may avoid being labeled or faulted for being "bad." Whether we perceive ourselves as "good" or "bad" becomes a matter of our identity—our ego. Be aware that there is a strong cultural propensity to romanticize "bad guys" in popular American tradition. If you find yourself identifying with the rebel, someone who likes to operate outside of the law or wanting to align with "badness," you may need to do some additional work to determine why you are identifying this and attempting to align in this manner. Did you have an early experience with an authority figure who acted inappropriately or unjustly? Have you carried this forward? Do your actions frequently stem from a seat of defiance? Who or what are you defying? These are a few questions to consider. Prepare to do some internal sleuthing and reflective thinking.

Authority figures and social systems do not always operate with individual vitality in mind. Maintaining an old pattern of behavior without regard to current situational appropriateness undermines our ability to use the system of the Four Gates to our physical advantage.

For example, continuing to act from a seat of defiance, as a result of circumstances long past or in reaction to an individual who is no longer part of our lives, impedes our personal progress and literally burns up our potential for achieving full vitality. With the original circumstances past or the offending individual gone, defiance and residual anger can actually turn us against our own internal authority—the essence or Self—and ultimately cause us to neglect or harm ourselves.

If you need help working through such an issue, do not be afraid to seek the assistance available through a competent, licensed professional. Remember this book is a limited resource and cannot take the place of the assistance provided by a competent professional.

From Judgment to Discernment

Long ago, there were once two neighbors living on the western edge of the far, far East. They had known each other for many, many years. After returning from a week-long trip, the first neighbor went to visit the second, who had remained home.

"You cannot imagine the difficulties I suffered upon your departure," the second neighbor groaned to the first. "Two of my prize stallions escaped into the night and out onto the steppe."

"Oh, that is awful," lamented the first neighbor in genuine sympathy with the second, "to lose two prize stallions in one night. What a terrible calamity."

"No, it is good!" exclaimed the stay-at-home neighbor. "My prize stallions each returned the next day with seven new beautiful mares. I now have fourteen additional horses," he said, clapping his hands together joyfully.

"That is indeed wonderful," smiled the first neighbor in agreement.

With his voice almost breaking, the second neighbor clenched his head. "No, it was terrible!"

"How can it be?" asked the first neighbor.

"You, better than anyone, know that I have too many children. My only son, the jewel of our house, was training one of the mares when the mare rolled on her side and broke my son's leg in four places. He will limp for the rest of his life," lamented the second neighbor.

"This is indeed a great misfortune," sympathized the first neighbor.

Exalted, the second neighbor shouted, "No, it is indeed good!"

"How can this be good, having your only son thus injured for the rest of his life?"

"I will tell you. That very weekend, the army came into the village and conscripted all eligible men. Because of his injuries, my precious gem was spared," exclaimed the first neighbor.

"It is indeed good," agreed the second neighbor, bowing to the first.

This Taoist teaching tale, a version of which may be found in Benjamin Hoff's book, *The Te of Piglet*,† illustrates how important it is to suspend judgment—even on events which seem like obvious setbacks. By urging us to take thoughtful steps away from our immediate reactions and encouraging us to wait to determine how an event may fit into the larger scheme of things, the tale invites us to create an observational stance. When we put off our most immediate emotional responses or reactions, our new, non-reactive cushion of safety allows us to shift—potentially—

† Please see pages 171-172 in the chapter, "Things as They Are."

From Judgment to Discernment

our point of view on a recent event. A setback may actually be an opportunity to lead a more authentic or meaningful life.

Making a shift from judgmental thinking to discernment is more than looking for the silver lining in a perceived cloud. By embracing discernment as a way of thinking and viewing life's events, we are capable of making a complete transformation in how we expend personal energy and precious time.

When discernment becomes our primary method of thinking and approach to the world, it allows us to live and revel more fully in the present than we may have been able to in the past. Discernment allows us to sharpen our focus and consolidate vital energy. With a fresh reserve of vital energy, we soon possess enough strength and resolve to make personally appropriate changes in our lives whenever we encounter situations that hinder growth, block our path or provide us with unexpected opportunities.

Discernment is careful consideration regarding decisions and details that concern and impact us directly—not someone else. In contrast to judgment, discernment is by nature an internal, self-reflective activity. Discernment possesses a healthy wait-and-see attitude. It is thoughtful. The shift from judgment to discernment, if we are tenacious, is a fairly straightforward one and may be accomplished using a few simple methods and techniques.

The first method of approach introduced here is the most direct in terms of helping us make a critical shift in thinking and eventually in behavior. Whenever we find ourselves beginning to form an opinion regarding something or someone else at hand, ask the question: Does this concern me directly? If it does not concern you directly, do not allow yourself to become involved. If a situation does seem to concern you directly, ask the next series of questions: What, if any, should my level of involvement be? What, if any, is my role in relationship to this situation or to this individual?

From Judgment to Discernment

Or, quite literally, what amount of my vital energy do I want to expend on this person or situation?[†]

When we do make a decision to become involved, the next step is to determine our level of involvement. How much energy do we intend to extend? If we do not have an ample supply of resources (e.g., compassion, organizational skills, time, expertise, funds) or a means by which we renew ourselves regularly, becoming involved in areas that do not concern us directly can be costly and depleting.[‡]

Participation in any situation may involve an expenditure of vital energy. Depending upon the

---

[†] If you are an intensely curious person, this habit of making inquiries into others' business can be difficult to break. Instead of attempting to suppress your innate curiosity, find another outlet for it by exploring other areas of interest. Make a trip to the library to begin researching other interests you have. In researching interests, you are also assisting your mind with its retooling process. You may even uncover new information that is appropriate to share at work or at home.

circumstances, we may recoup, lose or actually augment our personal energy. When choosing to involve ourselves in activities, situations or others' affairs, we benefit most by choosing relationships that foster personal growth and help us along our path rather than engaging in situations and relationships that prevent us from stepping onto our own unique path. So, the first act in shifting from judgment to discernment focuses on consolidating our personal energy.

Another approach to retooling the mind in order to make the shift from judgment to discernment works by means of calling ourselves into our present set of circumstances. It is an elegant observational tool, adapted from my days as a visual-arts graduate student, asking us to label what we are seeing or experiencing directly.

‡ The exception to this general rule occurs when people, who are in alignment, work with an organization or cause which has the greater good as its primary focus. Here too, the participants must have good personal boundaries in place in order to be effective and consistent as contributors.

From Judgment to Discernment

This exercise, in its generalized form, moves us into the body and heightens our awareness regarding our physical perceptions of the world around us in the present moment.

Thus, instead of allowing the mind to race aimlessly about on its own, forming opinions about whatever is at hand, we assign the mind observational tasks. These questions help us become grounded in our current circumstances. Here is the first option: What am I hearing, seeing, feeling, experiencing? Another option: What am I noting; how is my breathing; am I comfortable? Practicing in this manner, we automatically stop judgmental thinking and begin moving consciously into the body. With all of our vital energy moved into the body, we may begin observing our surroundings in a more pointed manner than we have in the past. Colors may seem brighter, sounds clearer and the edges of our visual experiences seem crisper.

After choosing one set of questions, repeat them to yourself when you are not actively engaged in another activity. Invite discernment into your mind by simply being fully aware of your current set of circumstances and enjoying or changing your immediate environment.

On occasion, there are situations where unplanned events may befall us, such as an unexpected sprained ankle as a result of a tumble down a steep, grassy slope. On the physical plane, sometimes things simply happen—unexplained and unannounced. In such circumstances, it is best to avoid pointing fingers or reliving an event over and over. Use your recovery time to look for positive possibilities in the situation. Is there a quiet project at home that has been waiting to be finished? Have you been wanting some time with a stack of favorite magazines or books? Is there anything new that you learned about yourself as a result of this occurrence? If the circumstances are more complex—perhaps involving a close friend or family member—and you yourself are not physically compromised, this may be your chance to assist someone else in need. In Sufism, it is said that behind every wounding there is a gift. Uncover it. The gift may be as simple as learning to receive or request help with humble gratitude.

Over time and after implementing these changes in thinking, you may notice a significant boost in your vitality. With your new reserve of energy, begin considering the twin questions: Who am I? And, why am I here? By shifting and then fine-tuning your thinking patterns, as well as working with the breathing exercises, important clues to these questions may begin to emerge.

Coming to Center: This breathing technique is traditionally taught in yoga classes after the body has been heated during a rigorous practice. From a physical point of view, it is designed specifically to cool the body. In my experience, the technique is also an expedient method of smoothing frayed emotions, as well as grounding the practitioner fully into the body.

Practice this technique when you are alone in your vehicle for a few minutes before shopping. This recommendation is made because it is a rare individual who has the luxury of carving out time at home for all of these exercises. Open the vehicle windows slightly for fresh air and lock the doors for safety. (If you do not own a vehicle, try this practice sitting upright on the edge of a chair, before bedtime or upon waking.)

Be sure to sit upright in order to gain maximum lung capacity. Think about breathing into your kidneys. You may also use a small, rolled towel at your lumbar curve in order to support your lower back—if you are leaning against your car seat or must lean against the back of a chair.

- Using fresh tissue, clear your nose until air is able to pass freely through both nostrils.

- Create a trough or straw with your tongue by rolling it into a tube. The tip of your tongue will jut out just past your parted lips.

From Judgment to Discernment

The trough allows cool air to pass through your mouth directly into your lungs. Approximately one in seven persons is unable to roll the tongue in this manner. If your tongue does not roll, simply place the middle of your tongue on your bottom lip with your lips parted slightly.

- Exhale through your cleared nose. Then, inhale through or over your tongue while counting slowly and steadily. Try working with a number between seven and twelve. When your lungs are comfortably full, remember the number you have reached while holding your breath in your lungs.

- As you begin counting anew, retract the tongue, close your mouth and lower your head toward your chest. Keep your breath in your lungs for the established count. Match your retention to that of your inhalation. †

- Next, using the established count, lift your head very slowly, expelling the air from your lungs through your nose. This is one smooth and fluid motion.

† Do not practice the retention if you have anxiety.

▪ As your lungs expand and the quality of your breath deepens, you may increase your count—even in this first sitting. The magic of the practice occurs when the count for inhalation, retention and exhalation are all of equal duration. *There should never be any discomfort or stress with this practice.* Hold the lungs comfortably full and without strain.

▪ Enjoy this exercise for three minutes, increasing the length of time to between five and seven minutes. Then, work up to twelve or fifteen minutes, if it feels appropriate.

Notes: In judging, we expend vital energy in making determinations regarding ourselves or others. Blaming and jealousy are forms of extended judgment. They too must be avoided. In blaming, we have already done the judging and continue to drain ourselves by faulting someone or something outside of ourselves. Blaming is, perhaps, the most costly emotional pattern or loop of which I am aware. As participants, it drains us of the very energy required to turn a situation around—or even turn ourselves around. Jealousy

From Judgment to Discernment

involves judging both another person (perhaps for having too much) and ourselves (perhaps for having too little) simultaneously. None of these behaviors leads to solutions in and of themselves. Judgment, blame and jealousy, as entrenched emotional patterns, sap us of our vital energy and should be avoided.

If you are unsure about whether or not you are losing vital energy to one of these patterns, do a self-check the next time you are walking down the street. Ask yourself several questions. Am I continuously observing and forming opinions about others' lifestyles, homes, clothing or bodies—especially unkind or non-complimentary ones? When you are involved in conversations at work, do you have a ready opinion or helpful "advice" on each topic at hand? Or, are you scrutinizing your own speech and behavior in such a way that the magnifying glass of judgment never leaves your own hand? If we find ourselves engaging with the world in any of these ways, reworking habituated thought patterns and processes will prove to be both helpful and, ultimately, calming.

■   ■   ■

There are two expressions in English that are in common parlance: "She exercises good judgment," and "He is a good judge of character." They describe a type of judgment which I would categorize as sound discernment. For the purposes of this chapter's discussion, judgment involves negative pigeon-holing, labeling and the formation of quick, ungrounded opinions about other individuals and their activities. Judgment may also involve your being overly harsh or critical toward yourself.

The one caveat I give in relationship to the discussion on judgment involves listening to gut instinct. Gut instinct may be described as a form of snap judgment, which I would categorize as comprehensive discernment, usually linked with a fight, flight or freeze response. Gut instinct is a sense to which you should pay close attention. If you find yourself walking in unfamiliar territory, while having an uneasy feeling, listen to yourself.

From Judgment to Discernment

If something inside of you says: "You need to shift to the other side of the street," or "I think that I need to take an alternate route home this evening," do not ignore this internal voice.

If you have experienced any trauma, sorting through your responses to the various stimuli of everyday living may prove to be difficult work. Please seek appropriate assistance from a trained, licensed professional who can help you directly.†

---

† The example that comes to mind involved my speaking with a veteran who was having difficulty embracing student night-life, after having returned from active combat. He had developed an acute degree of caution and wariness about going out after dark, while serving overseas, and was having difficulty setting aside this heightened, self-preserving behavior upon his return to civilian life.

Four Gates to Health

Two Consultants

Each of us is a unique blend of traits or characteristics, the combination of which renders us an entire personality. There are times when one discrete characteristic can take on a greater role than is typical. For example, if a situation triggers an unpleasant emotional response, we might find ourselves acting like a rebellious teenager. In an alternate situation, we surprise even ourselves when we handle a crisis with the calm of an emergency-response professional. For the purposes of this chapter's discussion, envision having only two aspects to the whole of your personality: a problem-solver and a creative consultant. These two aspects of ourselves are actually personifications of the left and right hemispheres of the brain. Our consultants know more about us than anyone else because they have been with us for our entire lives.†

This chapter is designed to help us tap the existing resources in our minds and live the constructive life available to us in present time. When properly applied, the concepts and practices also have the ability to draw us closer to center and the core of our essence—the Self.

Rediscovering critical aspects of our essential nature is a challenging process, requiring the marriage of skills exhibited by each of our hemispheres. For individuals who were blessed

† For further reading on hemispheric traits, see Dr. Jill Bolte Taylor's book, *My Stroke of Insight: A Brain Scientist's Personal Journey*. The text is accessible and her training is grounded in the Western medical model. Descriptions regarding the hemispheres' workings and traits mirror my own experiences.

with consistently supportive role models and balanced childhood experiences, this chapter's content may serve to polish skills we already employ without even thinking about them.

. . .

In one ideal, each of us would be born into a loving, supportive family, where our guardians would act as our primary guides or consultants in a sometimes complex and confusing world. In this scenario, the traditional twin, yogic questions—Who am I? And, why am I here?—would be entertained openly in the home. In childhood, our guardians, acting as our immediate role models, would openly pose these questions to themselves as adults and to us as children. We would then spend our time participating in a variety of activities, within a range of safe, diverse communities. We would discover our greatest strengths, as well as areas of interest and acumen, in a hammock of encouragement and ample supply. In short, we would uncover our personal best—our vital, grounded and centered Self. This is who we are at the level of essence. We are our personal best.

Some of us did not grow up in such a world and did not experience such a childhood. Instead of a nurturing childhood, some of us experienced overly taxed parents working diligently to supply us with our basic needs such as food, clothing and shelter. Others among us may have experienced parents foisting their own unrealized dreams upon us. In this scenario, we took lessons, played sports or studied things in which we showed no interest or sometimes even aptitude, while being told repeatedly how fortunate we were to receive such instruction.

In a home where one or both guardians continue to perceive theirs as a life of unrealized or broken dreams, the household often possesses a dark cloud of unresolved emotions. In such circumstances, an entire household may be haunted by disappointment, anger or bitterness. When these emotions accompany everyday living, even as an unspoken undercurrent, they detract from the joy, support and vitality available to the children growing up in that household.

Some of the most emotionally impoverished childhoods occur when we, as children, were told repeatedly that we were unwanted or made to feel like we were a burden. In a universal sense, such statements must be dismissed as untrue. And, if such statements were made to us as children, these statements do not warrant any further expenditure of vital energy on our part as adults. Such statements must be consciously and actively rejected, so that we do not waste additional vital energy on extended brooding, mourning, self-pity or in holding anger.

Consider yourself called here by a set of circumstances and power greater than those surrounding your family of origin. While it may be true that your family of origin was not ready for you, you were ready to be here. Consider life a learning mission. You owe it to yourself to become who you are. Remember that authority figures and institutions, when functioning, do not always have an individual's personal development and vitality in mind. You must work to enhance and safeguard your own vitality.

■ ■ ■

Imagine packing all of your less-than-optimal impressions and memories, from all phases of your life, into a box. In your mind's eye, seal that envisioned box and drop it into the ocean or burn it in a bonfire. Bring the full force of your focus squarely into your current set of circumstances. With the aid of your two, in-house consultants, you have an opportunity to implement positive changes in your life.

The first task involves sorting through your internal world. Start with a simple inventory. How do you talk to yourself when you are alone and there is no other information coming in? Are you encouraging and patient toward yourself? When reflecting, do you take time to give yourself sound, thoughtful advice? Are your thought patterns constructive in nature? Are you a kind and respectful problem-solver? If you find mostly unkind, critical words that are unconstructive directed toward yourself, it is time to supplant that former voice with the voice of your own new, custom-built and logical problem-solver.†

During the initial phases of this building process, consider carefully the primary qualities that you would like your problem-solver to exhibit. Your problem-solver may possess some of the same qualities that a favorite mentor exhibits toward you. Most of us desire a problem-solver who is compassionate, patient, understanding, wise and forgiving, while keeping us on task. We also appreciate a problem-solver who can offer sage, grounded advice, even as the rules of the world seem to be changing around us. If we are

---

† While in posture, I often ask my yoga students to speak internally to their own musculature. Students have noted that a harsh voice causes muscles to contract and perform poorly, while a calm and compassionate voice causes muscles to relax and outperform their requests. You may try this exercise yourself while stretching after your fitness routine.

Two Consultants

dreamy by nature, it is handy to have a problem-solver who develops a to-do list and keeps us on schedule. Be very sure and methodical when making this internal shift. Remember that discipline includes diplomacy and politeness. As your problem-solver begins to take shape, so too will the changed quality, tone, attitude and vocabulary in your mind. What should appear in your thoughts is the respectful voice of a linear-thinking, helpful and reliable mentor.

The activity of building a problem-solver causes you to establish an internal boundary. Being able to set boundaries, whether internal or external, is important for the success of your personal development. Learning to set this internal boundary will aid you in being able to set external boundaries later. Learning to set boundaries is part of being able to say "no" politely and resolutely or "yes" to things that increase your vitality. This critical, life skill will aid you as you restructure and refine your days. Be patient. We are all works-in-progress, beginning our work from the inside out. Think of your body and the space around your body as your own autonomous zone.

As you begin your retooling process, carefully monitor what you are exposing yourself to in terms of media, family contact and social gatherings. The initial phase of transition may be greatly hastened by selecting media and social circles that model the types of dialogue you want to hear in your own mind. Do not be afraid to skip movie night if the film being viewed is going to slow your progress during this process.† You deserve a better problem-solver. Do what you need to build and maintain one.   The initial transition requires time to take root, depending upon factors such as free time, exposure to appropriate models, childhood circumstances and the degree of contact you have with a supportive community.

† Even in ancient texts, such as *Narada's Bhakti Sutras,* there are recommendations for guarding an aspirant like the first tender shoot of a plant.

Two Consultants

Just as another person, in an exercise program participating alongside us, may serve as inspiration for our physical development, others—already speaking the way we would like to speak or behaving in a manner that we aspire to—may serve as role models or mentors for our personal growth.

Our progress may be accelerated when we choose to be among people who are positive and supportive of change, growth and vitality. If we do not have immediate support available, it is important to search for a group or set of individuals actively working on issues of self-improvement. For example, an organization that works on polishing public speaking skills may offer structured programming in which participants are encouraged to give and receive positive feedback, hone their voices or, potentially, work on the issue of reshaping personal story. Such an environment can be a safe, helpful and rewarding one for those of us working to grow and learn about ourselves.

Remember that membership in any group should be completely voluntary. There should be no penalty or repercussions at any time should you choose to leave a group. If at all possible, avoid contact with people who complain, blame or who are openly hostile. Such individuals may hinder progress during the early phases of building the ideal problem-solver consultant.

■   ■   ■

With our level-headed, problem-solver securely in place, we are now ready to rediscover our own creative consultant. This is the second phase of a two-part process. A stable problem-solver is critical to working with the creative consultant, who is more elusive and potentially shy due to issues of acculturation. Our society favors left-brain activities and systems, whether at school or at work. The problem-solver must be calm, trustworthy and supportive in order for the creative consultant to be invited out and made part of the consulting team.

■   ■   ■

If you have ever spent an afternoon with a group of small children, talking with them in a meaningful and thoughtful way, you know that, when trust is gained, children share the treasures of their hearts. Such treasures may be a collection of polished rocks, drawings of animals or some other cherished holding. It is that degree of trust we need to gain with ourselves, so that we may discover the things that are closest to our hearts—even as adults. This is the nature of the relationship we want in order to work successfully with our creative consultant and be able to uncover the desires of the heart.

The creative consultant is more tender and guarded than the problem-solver. How, then, do we work with our creative consultant? Most of our creative consultants share certain traits or qualities. Creative consultants are by nature spontaneous, enthusiastic, joyful, trusting, and emotionally honest. This is why having developed a consistent and trustworthy problem-solver is so critical to accessing and honoring the creative consultant. The creative consultant can help us uncover the desires of the heart. The heart is where joy resides.

If the world does not feel safe now or did not feel safe during childhood, our creative consultant may not be immediately or readily accessible. In addition to this, we are most likely unpracticed in processing and understanding our emotional impressions about our experiences. We may need professional help sorting through the relationship between our emotional impressions and our heartfelt desires, especially if our family's culture did not hold dear or value the things that we held dear as young children.

When first accessing the creative consultant, our environment must be safe. Begin this process when you are alone or with a very dear friend. Set aside short times for simply sitting quietly and watching your thoughts pass through your head like cloud formations. You choose which interesting cloud or idea to investigate based upon your own positive, internal emotional responses to them.

Another method of accessing the creative consultant is through movement. Day-to-day concerns surface and, then, release during the beginning of a walk, run or swim, creating space for fresh ideas to appear. During my own childhood, we engaged in automatic writing at school to clear away topical concerns, allowing us to access the essence of what we were intending to write for an assignment. Coloring and drawing work as well. It may feel forced or affected trying to access the right side of the brain through these exercises; but, it is worth remaining steady in our efforts because the creative consultant is the part of ourselves we must trust for fresh ideas and in recovering and while rediscovering the heart.

If you are encountering difficulties in determining whether or not you have forged a connection with your creative consultant, attempt a brainstorming session on free-time activities you would like to try. (If you are not adept at brainstorming, you may ask a trusted friend for assistance.) Brainstorming will become easier. Laughter, healthy play and free-form physical activities are additional means by which you can connect with this aspect of yourself.

The problem-solver sets the tone and parameters for meetings. The creative consultant comes up with ideas about the activities involved. Your left hemisphere is actually making an appointment with your right hemisphere. Here are a few examples of activities that your creative consultant might enjoy: swing in the park, play ball, lay in the sun or shade, collect stones, look at skateboards, go swimming, take a hike, read a book or watch someone get a tattoo. Think fun. Consider unusual. Start simply.

With creative consultants, the expressed desires rarely, if ever, involve extravagant expenditures. Expensive taste comes with social awareness. Your creative consultant enjoys simple pleasures and wants to spend time with you while engaged in fun activities that are in alignment with your essence and boost your vitality. Thus, the creative consultant is not about status or ostentatious display. The creative consultant is about how you spend your time. Be kind to your Self. Ensure that you feel well cared for, by being a good listener and treating yourself with patience and gentle kindness.

Here is an example on how to integrate these ideas and practice them in daily life. Imagine it is a Saturday. You started your morning by withdrawing funds that you budgeted for the day's purchases. During the course of the day, you stood in line at the post office, went grocery shopping and found exceptional discount athletic shoes for your children. It is the end of the day.

You are tired and hungry. Your childcare provider is not expecting you for another two hours. You decide to treat yourself to a solo, sit-down dinner at the local southwestern restaurant. While you are headed into the restaurant, you open your wallet to determine your budgetary limit. What you find is that the twenty dollars you had set aside was spent on two extra ingredients at the grocery store. Crestfallen, you wend your way back through the parking lot. You are tired and hungry, but it is time to regroup. This is when the steady voice of the problem-solver steps in asking, "Would you like to get take-out tacos and eat in the park?" You have a few dollars left and enough change.

The answer to this question is "yes." We may not be able to enjoy the full, sit-down meal experience, but there is still sustenance and leisure to be enjoyed in the second option. Take the second option. In time, it may even become the option of choice. It is how we spend time, talk with and treat ourselves that matters. And, as with everything, it is a balancing act.

Here are some simple guidelines for continuing your work. As you build your ability to connect and dialogue with your two consultants, you will also be able to work, in a limited way, with some issues from childhood.

Two Consultants

Most of us live with a few unrequited childhood desires. Maybe you thought that you wanted a dog. To resolve this unmet desire, as an adult, you may decide to enroll in a volunteer experience allowing you to work with dogs. After a series of lessons in volunteering, you find out that working with dogs is not as much fun as you thought it would be. Maybe you even discover that you have a moderate allergy that you did not know about. Suddenly, that used trail bike on sale in the bicycle shop is what you really would like to try on the trails outside of town. Rent or buy a used one first. Working with this practice in an expanded format can help us resolve some of our unrequited childhood desires. Take care to look after your consultants and the desires of your heart. Following is an illustrative story about maintaining watch over your heart.

. . .

Once, in speaking with a gentleman about one of my writing projects, I was surprised when he began asking me very detailed questions about a local writing group. He did not appear to be a person who would be interested in any sedentary activity. My face became quizzical.

In way of explanation regarding his inquiry, he stated, "I found out that my wife has been writing. Can you believe that she has been hiding it from me? She was afraid to tell me that she was even interested in writing."

Writing must be at a very tender, new stage for this woman and close to her heart. Perhaps writing was an unrealized childhood dream, for which she received little or no encouragement. When we first uncover our deepest desires, they are tender and new. Sometimes we must guard our desires from the people who are closest to us because those closest to us may not understand or be fully supportive of our dreams.

If you are concerned about sharing your heart's desires with someone close, you have given that person too much power—to support or not support you with their words or other actions. Reclaim your power over your volition.

Two Consultants

In the previous example, although this woman was much loved and enjoyed a supportive relationship with her husband, she did not want any feedback because even doubtful feedback might have destroyed her connection to her nascent volition in this area. Do not grant another individual or group that much power over your decision-making ability, creativity or heart. Then, when you are ready, find a supportive group of like-minded individuals, who deliver constructive feedback, to help foster your development or, alternately, help you release an outmoded desire. Any outcome is possible. Your problem-solver and creative consultant have a safe haven in your own body. Work to strengthen your physical body and create a sanctuary for the entirety of your sacred essence.

Balancing Both Hemispheres: This exercise is patterned after the alternate-nostril breathing of yogic tradition. Because we are born into the world on the wave of the first breath, and we leave the world on the crest of our last breath, Eastern healing traditions often consider our respiratory system the body's first system of digestion and its primary source of nourishment.

This practice is offered here to help balance the functional operation of both hemispheres of your brain. Think of this technique as rejuvenating for your consultants. Practiced regularly, alternate-nostril breathing seems to promote clear, grounded and balanced thinking. Additional descriptions about how to practice this technique are found in most comprehensive books on yoga.

Practice this technique in your parked vehicle, with locked doors, before or after work—or during a lunch break. Again, the recommendation for using your vehicle is made because it is a rare individual who has the luxury of space or time to practice this method at home. If there is a safe, green space nearby, practice there. The technique may also be practiced in a seated position at the edge of a chair in your home. Have fresh tissue at hand to clear your nose.

▪ Place your left hand, palm down, to rest on your left thigh. Your index finger should touch your thumb, making an okay symbol with your left hand. Your left elbow hangs comfortably directly below your shoulder.

▪ Place your right-hand index and middle fingers between your eyebrows. Form a backward letter "C," using your ring finger and thumb. Allow your little finger to follow the curve of your ring finger. Your elbow falls toward your navel. (Alternately, you may curl your index and middle fingers toward the center of your palm.)

▪ With your right hand, place your thumb and ring finger just below the bone in your nose. Take turns closing off alternate nostrils, breathing through the open side. You may notice that one side of your nose is easier to breathe through than the other.

▪ The side through which you can breathe most freely is the active side. The more (perhaps) congested side is your passive side. If you are a person blessed with a consistently clear nose, assign the role of active side to your right nostril and that of the passive side to your left nostril.†

▪ With tissue at hand, blow your nose to clear the congested side. After clearing, you should be able to work some degree of air through the passive side without straining. If you have a cold or flu, practice this exercise on another day.

▪ Sitting tall, empty the lungs completely with an exhaling breath. Next, take a full, even breath through both sides of your nose.

▪ Close the passive side and exhale through the active side. Next, close the active side and inhale through the passive side. Your hand shifts from side to side as you close off the side opposite from the called breath. Exhale active. Inhale passive. Exhale active. Inhale passive.

† If you have chronically congested sinuses, you might consider consulting a healthcare professional or dietician to determine whether or not you have any chronic, low-grade food allergies, or you may consider investing in a neti pot.

Two Consultants

• Now, keeping the active side closed, exhale on the passive side. Inhale on the active. Exhale passive. Inhale active. Exhale passive. Inhale active. Finish by exhaling through both nostrils.

• The bridge of the nose remains steady as you work. Closing the nostrils is a subtle movement that does not involve shifting the cartilage about. Your breath is subtle, comfortably expansive and even. Be gentle.

• For the purposes of this book, this is considered one cycle of the breathing pattern. In one ideal, this technique would be practiced for three cycles, two to three-times daily.

• Rather than emphasizing the number of times daily or number of cycles to be practiced at one sitting, I have found it helpful to focus on reaching a point where I am able to breathe freely through both nostrils for a final set of three full cycles.

• This breathing technique is a great boon in the late afternoon, when there is a natural dip in our energy.

• Here is the short-hand version of the practice you completed. Experiment with the two additional patterns included here.

Empty your lungs with one slow, thorough exhaling breath.

Inhale through both sides of the nose.

Exhale active	Inhale passive
Exhale active	Inhale passive
Exhale active	Inhale passive
Exhale passive	Inhale active
Exhale passive	Inhale active
Exhale passive	Inhale active

Exhale through both sides of the nose.
Resume normal breathing on the inhale.

Empty your lungs with one slow, thorough exhaling breath.
Inhale through both sides of the nose.

Exhale passive	Inhale passive
Exhale passive	Inhale passive
Exhale passive	Inhale passive
Exhale active	Inhale active
Exhale active	Inhale active
Exhale active	Inhale active

Exhale through both sides of the nose.
Resume normal breathing on the inhale.

Two Consultants

Empty your lungs with a slow, thorough exhaling breath.

Inhale through both sides of the nose.

Exhale passive	Inhale passive
Exhale active	Inhale active
Exhale passive	Inhale passive
Exhale active	Inhale active
Exhale passive	Inhale passive
Exhale active	Inhale active

Exhale through both sides of the nose.

Resume normal breathing on the inhale.

Hint: Here are several tips for working with the issue of chronic congestion.

Option One: If the right nostril remains congested, turn your head completely to the right and practice as many cycles of breathing as necessary until that side clears. Likewise, if the left side is congested, turn your head to the left and practice as many cycles of breathing as necessary until the left side clears.

Option Two: Place a tennis ball in the armpit *opposite* the side of congestion. Hold the tennis ball securely in your armpit without straining, using your arm and chest muscles to press it into the side of your body as you wait for the congested side to clear.

Option Three: If you do not have a tennis ball, you may use your fist. For example, if your right nostril is congested, make a fist with your right hand and place it comfortably in your left armpit in lieu of the tennis ball. You may choose to begin the practice with this option.

Note: On occasion, we may find ourselves crushed by means of our own harshness—without any outside aid at all. This phenomenon may be a carry-over from childhood if we lacked emotional support, felt powerless or were treated harshly by our caregivers or peers. If at some point feeling disappointed became our internal, emotional norm, newfound joy or happiness may cause us to experience a sense of suspicion or guilt, as though contentment is an unnatural state. The breathing practices will aid you in resetting your internal, emotional markers.† Be patient and consistent in your practice of these techniques. Allow calm contentment to enter your body and help you build vitality.

Ultimately, we are looking to come to center in the present in order to experience joy and contentment in a more holistic manner than previously imagined possible.

† Excepting cases of clinical consideration, which are outside the scope of this book, a state of consistently mild, internal disappointment may be addressed through the appropriate application of the featured breathing practices.

From a Seat of Graciousness

Drawing closer to operating from our own unique center sometimes causes us to experience a jarring realization. Our most immediate world—close friends, social networks, co-workers and family—may no longer feel like a good fit. In coming to center, former patterns of choice, behavior and relationship, which were once desirable or comfortable sometimes lose their luster. We may even discover that once favorite touchstones of humor are no longer funny. Formerly comfortable patterns of relationship may begin to feel less-than-optimal—even if family and friends have begun transformational work of their own.

How do we maintain our newly established center in an unchanged external world—or, in reality, in our ever-changing external world? While we may experience a pronounced desire for immediate change in our environment or a change in the behavior from those around us, we can only work on changing ourselves. We cannot do others' internal or transformational work for them. We cannot save or protect others from what we perceive to be their own less-than-optimal behavior. In order to safeguard and maintain our newly established center, we must learn to operate from a seat of graciousness.†

Gracious behavior, which is sometimes considered one of life's extras, is actually critical to

---

† One major consideration for most students at this point is whether or not they want to remain in the context of established relationships. In lecture, the importance of safe, supportive relationships for personal growth is stressed. If you find yourself in a relationship where personal safety is in question, seek professional guidance for additional assistance.

Four Gates to Health

personal growth. Gracious behavior promotes upliftment, expansion and a strengthening of the essence which, in turn, causes us to gain vitality and start the process of charting our very individual course from a seat of strength. Finally, gracious behavior, in speech and action, aids us in disentangling ourselves from the imbalances inherent in many of our existing relationships.

While our fitness program continues to help us resolve issues of strength and stamina on the outside, application of the concepts, breathing practices and gracious behavior help hold us steady on the inside. We interface with our family, peers and co-workers through our speech and actions. Ideally, operating from a seat of graciousness assists our process of development, unfolding and thriving, allowing us to continue unhindered by our most immediate community. By adding gracious behavior to the skills you already have in place, you may experience an outward shift toward a more authentic life that is consistent with your essence. Let us look at making some additional changes.

For many of us, our daily manner of speaking and interacting with others stems from a series of preconditioned behavioral patterns that were modeled in our earliest years and environments or from places of injury to our hearts. Stepping away from preconditioned patterns of response is extremely challenging work. While this is true, it is also true that working to change our social behavior is worth all of the effort we put into it. In stepping away from preconditioned responses, we are finally able to speak and act in thoughtful ways that are consistent with the authentic and compassionate strength of our essence.

Our disambiguated essence, coupled with pure intention, is the powerhouse of personal integrity. When we become practiced in making decisions and acting from a seat of graciousness and the space of our hearts, *we are able to affirm our own vitality without compromising another's*. We will begin relating and operating, in the context of community, in ways that we may not have attempted before or even imagined possible. Through our heightened observational skills, we become increasingly aware of social intricacies, others' feelings and the results of our own actions or lack of action. This new awareness grants us multiple opportunities to act more consistently from the space of our hearts. Before presenting the primary model for operating from a seat of graciousness, let us look at a classic tale about a reactive household.

In this tale, the reactive pattern of behavior is set off by an adult parent, male or female, who is unable to process personal emotions after a very difficult day at work. Upon arriving home, the emotionally frustrated parent verbally reprimands the oldest child without due cause. The oldest child who is hurt, confused and angry about being yelled at for no logical reason, then yells at a younger sibling. The younger sibling passes the invisible ball of disruptive, unresolved emotion—originally from the parent—onto the youngest sibling by snatching away a toy. Finally, the youngest child might pass the snowballed frustration onto the family pet by behaving unkindly toward that innocent family member.

Looking at this scenario from the outside, it is easy to see that one invisible, unresolved mass of emotion set the entire family into a tailspin. Everyone is reacting without thinking, perpetuating emotional chaos and pain. In this scenario, no one in the household knows how to do anything but react to what is openly emoted. Fortunately, there are other options—more personally and socially productive ones. We have the power and ability to behave differently from the ways in which we may have been expected or shown to behave. I say "may have been shown" purposefully because it is possible for a gracious household to have a reactive child, and it is possible for a reactive household to have a gracious child. In both circumstances the question then becomes one of potential learning.

Four Gates to Health

76

In Vedic theory, an individual soul may actually carry forward both desirable and undesirable aspects of personality from previous incarnations. The undesirable traits must then be worked through, mitigated or resolved in successive incarnations. This does not excuse an individual soul from taking responsibility for less-than-optimal speech or actions in a given lifetime. Such souls must put forth even greater effort to transform themselves over the course of a single lifetime or series of lifetimes. Nonetheless, through self-awareness, discipline, behavior modification and the release of ego, "liberation" of a soul is possible in the context of a single lifetime.

Before proceeding, take a moment to recall two questions that apply in any situation: Does this concern me directly? And, what amount of vital energy, if any, do I want to expend on this situation? Using these two questions before speaking or acting helps us avoid openly reacting even when another individual may solicit this type of response from us by delivering an emotional hook.† Remain an observer until you have time to determine what role, if any, you want to play. Avoid allowing someone else to wind you up emotionally and tap you energetically. If you do choose to engage, know that you are in fact giving away something of yourself when you participate.

In terms of preventing ourselves from reacting, what we need to be aware of is an unwarranted amount of rising emotion inside of ourselves. If strong emotions begin to rise, observe and acknowledge them internally ("I am feeling...." "Or, I am experiencing..."), and then, attempt to exhale those emotions right out. Sometimes a vigorous run or walk is required. Internally, take a moment to determine why the situation or individual is warranting a heightened

---

† Individuals who deliver information with a heightened degree of emotion attached to it may be enjoying a false high while riding the roller coaster of their own emotions and perceived life drama. Such personalities, if they can hook others, seem to thrive on sharing their reactivity.

emotional response. It may be that a childhood or life-changing memory was triggered. Be patient. Pause and sort through possible causes for your excessive emotional response before adding your own emotions or reactivity to a situational mix. Continue to ask yourself: Does this concern me directly? And, what amount of vital energy, if any, do I want to expend on this situation? Deciding to remain a calm observer causes us to conserve our vitality, avoid misunderstandings and miscommunications, as well as helping us take the first steps toward developing a consistently gracious demeanor.

· · ·

There are two minimum requirements for operating from a seat of graciousness. The first requirement is sincere effort. Stepping away from our preconditioned responses is highly demanding work—especially if we are used to being surrounded by reactive personalities. We must become scrupulously self-aware, observant, quiet, forgiving and tenacious in our efforts to change the ways in which we automatically behave. We are most vulnerable to falling into old patterns when we are tired, hungry or distracted. The second critical component in making lasting changes has to do with our willingness and ability to unearth and relinquish the beliefs or notions that hold our habituated behaviors in place.

Behind almost every deeply emotional reaction there is a notion or belief about the nature of the world and the way things work (*i.e.,* People are out to get one another. People are basically good, only a little misguided. If I don't say "yes," that person won't like me.). Unexamined, fixed notions often keep us from operating from the expansiveness of our own essence and the strength of our hearts, where graciousness resides.

When we find ourselves experiencing greater emotional responses than a given situation warrants, whether our emotions are expressed outwardly or not, we must trace our responses back to the experience, belief system or notion that holds the root of our reactivity in place. This process requires tenacious self-examination and excavation. Once the experience or notion is uncovered, acknowledge it. And, then, make a conscious decision about whether or not you will let go of it. Releasing the emotions attached to old experiences and fixed notions is the fastest way to move toward enhanced vitality and emotional freedom. Work on developing your ability to view your world from an observational stance with an open, non-judgmental mind. All of your enhanced ability to discern should be trained upon learning about yourself, how you want to interact, live and what relationships you would like to foster or develop.

Fortunately for us, the act of living is replete with opportunities for practicing graciousness. Take small steps as you make adjustments to your own behavior and attitudes toward your immediate community.   Try implementing the model outlined below until you have gained self-assurance and humble confidence.

For consistency and convenience, the initial phase for operating from a seat of graciousness is outlined using a scenario similar to the first, with slightly altered parameters and outcomes. As you may recall, in our tale of a family in a fixed reactive pattern, it was the parent who set things in motion by being unable to process emotions left over from a difficult day at work. In the last few pages, the parent has neither become involved in transformational work nor has the parent made other progress. The oldest child, however, has completed a parenting skills course and psychology class in school. The oldest child has a new awareness on behavioral issues and options. In the second scenario, only the oldest child is home when the parent returns from work with a menacing cloud of unresolved emotion.

Upon coming home, the parent verbally rebukes the oldest child for no apparent reason.

Seeing that the parent has had a bad day and that the parent's rebuke has nothing to do with his or her own behavior, the oldest child decides the best thing to do is to leave the situation. The child gives the parent some time alone by saying, "I am going next door to do homework with Jonathan. Here is his number. Call me before dinner, and I will come home to set the table."

In this scenario, the child is acting from a seat of graciousness by caring for his or her own vitality and essence first. (This idea is similar to the advisory given on airplanes: In the event that the oxygen masks deploy, place your mask on first, before assisting those around you, including children.) The child has surmised that the situation at home will not be made better by remaining at home. By choosing to act in a preemptory manner, the child gives the parent both space and time to process and, hopefully, regain some degree of emotional equilibrium. Learning to separate ourselves from others' emotions grants us the opportunity to observe situations and take actions that are most appropriate for our short- and long-term vitality.†

Thus, in this initial model for operating from a seat of graciousness, we are involved in learning to honor our own vitality. By using our heightened abilities to observe our surroundings and being able to read situations with greater clarity than before, we are capable of taking respectful, self-preserving action. Ideally, this would happen *before* anything which might cause us serious

† Some may view this second scenario as regrettable, where a child is expected to employ gracious behavior toward a dysfunctional adult. In such a case, a child is forcibly cast into the role of adult or parent. Nonetheless, all of us, at some point, find our roles reversed with greater frequency than we might desire. At work, for example, there are individuals, holding positions of authority over us, who require those under their functional jurisdiction to act as their emotional stewards. Such situations are training grounds for learning how to set appropriate boundaries, behave graciously and/or invite us to make personal changes; thereby, assisting us in the greater scheme of things with the issue of coming into alignment with the Self.

harm or significant pain. This is where and why the breathing exercises become so critical. In addition to promoting internal awareness, the breathing exercises help us learn to read the subtleties of various circumstances and social situations with greater skill and accuracy than before. Honoring our own vitality aids us in building energetic reserves. These reserves help us accumulate the vitality required to develop fortitude, nourish our observer and become clear and diplomatic in our transactions with others.

In this model for gracious behavior, we are learning to care for our own essence—without harming others. This model is not about selfishness, self-indulgence or the sustaining of false stories to which our egos cling. Gracious behavior is about minding the sanctity of the Self. If you have been brought up in a home where your body, vital energy or essence were not honored, or where you were unable to set personal boundaries for your own health and safety, practicing this initial step may feel unnatural and awkward. You may even experience guilt while honoring some of your basic needs. Know that this first step, the honoring of the Self, is necessary to progress.

As you may recall, when working with the two hemispheres of the brain, we set a boundary with our own, sometimes harsh, internal voice in order to develop the voice of our problem-solver consultant. Much of the work around developing gracious behavior actually requires us to learn how to set and maintain personal, vitality-enhancing boundaries. In way of definition, personal boundaries are the parameters for living which we set for ourselves or, perhaps, for the small children for whom we care. One example of setting a boundary might involve saying "no" to an old friend who wants us to participate in an activity that we have since learned saps us of vital energy. Another example may involve telling our domestic partner that we need to go to bed earlier, sleep later or begin our morning by taking the first shower, so we have more personal time before work. Setting boundaries involves politely outlining specific requirements we must follow in order to maintain our health and well-being. We are, in fact, saying yes to our own essence.

When setting a boundary, it is best to think in terms of saying "yes" to activities and choices that are life enhancing. For example, committing to making Wednesday afternoon our time-at-the-fitness-center honors the body. Honor yourself and begin rearranging your days, so that you experience a zest for life and new sense of freedom. Rearranging the details of your days and setting boundaries will soon become an automatic and natural part of your daily routine.

Remember there are two consultants at your beck and call, as well as the breathing practices, to help you resolve any apparent roadblocks or questions you may encounter. The creative consultant is adept at brainstorming solutions, while the problem-solver keeps you grounded and on task. Dedication to your fitness program and the breathing practices will continue to enhance your strength and sense of self-reliance as you gain vital energy and awareness.

A few of my students have asked, "What are some of the results of becoming consistently gracious?" One of the most wonderful things that I have observed happen, when we begin to function from a seat of graciousness, is that we find ourselves among new friends. We are able to begin associating with individuals who also operate behaviorally to the benefit of their own and, then, include considerations of others' well-being. Finally, when an entire community begins functioning from a seat of graciousness, we have the potential to create a web of healthier relationships on an ever-expanding scale.

Walking Breath: This exercise is a real boon to those who enjoy movement-based practices. It stands as a point of contrast to the seated and reclining practices, which can dominate Eastern schools of contemplative learning. Before setting out, be sure that you have an excellent pair of walking shoes, to wear in a safe neighborhood, comfortable socks and a clear nose. Pay attention to the length and position of your spine in space. As you walk, lift your breastbone, along with your rib cage, so that you create ample space for the whole of your middle torso. Your head, neck, upper body and moving arms float above your legs and hips as you walk.

- After clearing your nose, begin with an exhale. Engage your abdominal muscles and envision releasing stale air from each corner of your lungs and all parts of your body.

- On an inhaling breath, begin counting as you fill your lungs comfortably and fully with fresh, outside air.

- Match the count of your exhalation to that of your initial inhalation. Repeat this even breathing pattern for seven cycles. You may feel an expansiveness in your rib cage that you have not experienced before.

- Next, after inhaling naturally to your established count, retain the breath in the lungs for a quarter of your full count. For example, if you are inhaling to eight and exhaling to eight, you would then inhale for eight, retain the breath in the lungs for two counts and resume exhaling for eight. Follow this pattern for seven cycles of breathing.

▪ Now, pause to check in with your body. Are you beginning to feel enlivened? If any discomfort or light-headedness occurs, take a break from this practice and return to your normal breathing.

▪ If the first portion of this exercise was grounding and invigorating, you may choose to retain the breath in the lungs, after your inhalation, for half of your full count. Following the example given above, the shorthand would look like this: Inhale for a count of eight, retain for four and exhale for eight. Next, complete seven additional cycles of breathing using this new pattern.

▪ If walking—as an activity—is new to you, or breath-based practices are new, please enjoy just this much of the practice for one outing. Spend the remainder of your time on the walk observing the details of your outside environment. Focus on small things. There is beauty in the small, overlooked details of life.

▪ If you are a seasoned walker and have been working through the breath-based practices in this book, you will now decrease the time that you retain the breath in the lungs to one quarter of your established count. Using the example from the previous paragraphs, the shorthand would be—inhale for eight, retain for two and exhale for eight. Do this for seven additional cycles.

▪ In the final phase, step the count down. Your inhalation will match your exhalation, with no retention. Use this breathing pattern for as long as it feels comfortable in your body. Return to normal breathing should you begin to tire.

Note: If you were raised in a reactive household, do not waste additional vital energy on blaming your family of origin or guardians for your current circumstances. The individuals who raised you could not model alternate behavioral patterns because they themselves were untrained in alternate methods of relating to the world. One

From a Seat of Graciousness

method of approaching past injuries involves being grateful, in current time, for finding alternate models of behavior and then actively implementing the new models. Focus on keeping all of your awareness and energy in present time.

If you are still having difficulty releasing past circumstances, you must formally address the issue of forgiveness. Forgiving the past and then releasing it is the most efficient method of moving toward emotional freedom and forward with transformation. Internally, make statements of forgiveness until you feel the heaviness about that relationship, circumstance or issue lift from your chest. Read your breath. You will know you have successfully forgiven the past when you are able to speak diplomatically about your past circumstances, those who raised you and other apparent setbacks with gratitude.

Eventually, you may create an alternate support system or "new family" to help you continue on your personal journey.

Resilience

One afternoon, as class was beginning, one of my most genuine students approached me with an inquiry. "Do you follow your horoscope?" It was an inquiry that caused me a moment of internal mirth. When I looked into her face, I realized her question was quite serious. Not wanting to be disrespectful or hurt her in any way, I paused to reflect on the possible questions underlying her spoken words. Where do you go when you are seeking guidance? Or, where should I go when I am seeking guidance? The issue of seeking guidance concerns all of us at some point.

Before taking up one possible answer to this student's inquiry, let's revisit the primary assumption underlying this book. We have made a commitment to consolidating and enhancing personal vitality by choosing to participate in a fitness program. Our fitness program takes into consideration such factors as age, gender, body type and issues of accommodation for preexisting physical concerns. Our program is neither a source of pain to be endured nor an exercise in unhealthy excessiveness or extremes. Ideally, there is also enough quiet time built into our fitness routine or into the time spent on the breathing techniques that we are able to listen to the body in a way we may not have been able to listen before. In Eastern terms, our fitness program is our physical practice.

The second assumption underlying this book is that we have a commitment to discovering who we are at our personal best. When we honor ourselves by engaging in regular, healthy activities and habits, we may become resilient.

Listening to the wisdom of the body, when we are in alignment with the heart, is the most critical life skill that we can develop to enhance our vitality. Listening to the body involves not only noticing an uncomfortable knee or pinching elbow, but it means observing how the body responds to various stimuli—whether the stimuli are the foods we eat, the entertainment we select, the vocational or avocational activities we practice or how we schedule the events and obligations of our days. By learning to read the body, we have the ability to make concrete lifestyle changes and adjustments, so that we may begin to thrive. Let's look at one scenario about learning to read the body and, by extension, becoming more resilient.

In this scenario, you choose to view a newly released film in a movie theater. Near the end of the film, you develop a mild headache. Perhaps the volume in the theater was too high, the seats were misaligned, causing you to strain to see, or the treats you chose were inappropriate. Upon arriving home, you decide to make some adjustments to your movie routine, possibly opting for a stay-at-home movie night so that you control the volume, arrange your own seating and enjoy snacks that are better for your body. In another variation on this scenario, you decide that you cannot do without the big-screen experience. To mitigate the possibility of another headache, you decide to use earplugs, choose a better seat and forego the in-house treats. Whatever decisions you make, remember to stay attuned to your body for feedback, mark the quality of your breath and listen to the wisdom of your essence for cues on how to proceed.

There is an additional concept that bears consideration at this point in our discussion. *Coincidence is not necessarily an indicator of causality.* In light of the movie scenario, it may be that the mild headache you developed had nothing to do with the hypothesized factors but was actually due to the first stages of a common cold. The more attuned you are, to your body, breath and environment, the easier it becomes to determine how you should proceed. Remember, you may not always find the cause or causes for certain of your discomforts. A sense of adventure and humor can help keep the process of discovery light and place things in perspective.

In the second scenario, we are looking at a more complex situation than we reviewed previously. Let's assume you have made adjustments in your lifestyle so that you are feeling more alive and vital than ever before. One day, you receive a catalogue in the mail from the local community college offering noncredit evening classes. With all of your newfound energy, you decide to look through the listings and try a class. You may even make some new friends. You enroll for a six-week course, which meets twice weekly in the late evening for ethnic cooking, or you might choose another listing that appeals to your imagination.

The first class that you attend is fun and interesting. You are open to possibilities. As time lapses, your initial enthusiasm wears off. But you cannot determine the exact cause for your loss of interest. Remember, this is a noncredit, voluntary activity at a reasonable cost. Soon lack of enthusiasm turns to dread.

By the beginning of the fourth week, you can barely make yourself get out of the house to attend the last few classes. Mentally, you run through possible reasons for wanting to quit. Your classmates are not the people you had hoped to meet. The food is not to your taste. The time of day is wreaking havoc with your sleep cycles—so much so that you are tired at work. Eating ethnic food is great but ethnic food preparation is tedious. Yours and the instructor's personalities are not a good fit. Or, the adhesive under the newly laid tile floor in the community-college kitchen is still outgassing and taxing your body. No matter what the reason may be, every fiber of your body is telling you to stop attending.

This experience is one of learning. Listen to your body. Let go. Stop attending. It is perfectly acceptable to leave a situation if it is harmful to you. Life is full of additional opportunities.

Modern living presents a number of circumstances in which reading the body for feedback becomes challenging. In situations where unseen environmental factors may have an adverse impact on the body (*e.g.*, exposure to toxic chemicals in new building materials or higher-than-normal levels of radiation exposure from a series of medical tests) and for those suffering from autoimmune diseases, it can be challenging to sort out exactly what makes us feel fatigued, short-tempered or unwell. Nonetheless, the body is the instrument through which we experience the world and the vessel in which we live our lives. At some point, excepting serious psychological or medical concerns, it is the body and the quality of the breath that we must rely on for feedback and, ultimately, our decisions.

It is important to take time to sort through our circumstances and dialogue with the body during the practice of our breathing exercises or fitness routine. The body offers insights, hints and clues about how to proceed with decisions and take action. By observing the body and the breath throughout the day, we may respond, if needed, by making changes to our schedule. By learning to read the body and the quality of the breath in this way, most of our days will present themselves as ever-unfolding moments filled with wonder and increasing joy.

While charting our life course, there are times when we come across individuals so radiant and at the peak of performance that we want to know the secret behind their success. Turn an observant pair of eyes and ears to others and their stories. Personal biography can be one of the most efficient methods of learning about others' varied paths to personal fulfillment. At the same time, remember that you have your own course to set and the seeds of your own garden inside. Be especially aware and even wary of individuals and organizations that promise immediate, extraordinary material gain as part of their program of advancement. Life is a balancing act and personal fulfillment may not be linked to material gain. With that stated, know that those who feel a sense of fulfillment, because they are in alignment, often describe feeling wealthy—whether or not they have experienced a gain in material wealth. A sense of fulfillment comes from honoring the essence—the Self. Something as simple as a change in geographic location, work schedule, vocation, attitude or social group can assist us in enhancing our vitality, as well as honoring the essence of being.

Let's return now to the issue of seeking guidance. Many false starts and a few metaphorical stops have caused me to pay close attention to the wisdom of my body. While engaged in my fitness routine or daily breathing exercises, I take time to listen carefully to the feedback my body and breath provide, keeping the focus on my most immediate concerns. The system of the Four Gates has allowed me to resolve the majority of my dietary and activity concerns with greater ease. Years of practice with the system of the Four Gates, my body and breath have taught me how to make ever more appropriate personal choices. Over time, I have rearranged priorities, scheduling and relationship commitments based upon what my body and breath have "said." Your body and breath are the quickest, surest ways to seek and receive guidance. Learn to become mindful of them, and you will be able to receive answers about how to proceed through each unique day.

Thus, the guidance we seek is available to us by going within. The oracle does not reside outside—in a horoscope column, with a peer group, in the body responses or psychological experiences of another person—but inside of ourselves. While it is true that there are circumstances when it is important to converse with others about alternate perceptions and perspectives, eventually we must find our own answers and wholeness inside. After completing your daily breathing practice, listen and wait for answers to your own questions, posing only those questions which concern you directly. Continue consolidating your personal energy by remaining focused on your own fitness routine, behavior, activities and path. The wisdom of the body in alignment with the essence should yield answers to your inquiries. The essence rides the breath. Your awareness of the unique rhythm of your essence will allow you to listen to the subtle voice of your heart and that of your true Self.

Uncovering the Essence: This foundational breathing practice is normally used during the practice of yoga's physical postures. It is essential for uncovering who we are at the level of essence. In Sanskrit, the breathing technique is sometimes referred to as conquering or conqueror's breath. In English, it is sometimes called ocean-sounding breath. You do not have to attend a yoga class to gain the many benefits from this practice. Use this technique while walking, bicycling or gardening. Imagine being able to achieve runner's high while washing your car or mopping the kitchen. This method of breathing is that powerful. Before taking a walk with this technique, practice while sitting tall on the front half of a chair.

- Extend your index fingers and place them gently below the jaw line in the natural space, where the front of the throat merges with the side of the neck. There should be a natural indentation or hollow.

- Open your mouth. Create a small constriction at the top of your throat, exhaling the "H" sound through your mouth. The sound is said to be reminiscent of the ocean waves. You may also think of the throat action as being the same as the one used when fogging a mirror with your breath.

- Keeping your mouth open and throat gently constricted, inhale "H" through your mouth. Think about reaching down to your toes, into your fingers and to your crown on the inhaling breath. If your climate is not overly dry, practice three full rounds of breathing the "H" while holding your mouth open.

• Next, remove your index fingers from below the jaw line while retaining the constriction at the top of the throat. Gently close your mouth and continue exhaling and inhaling "H" through your nose. Your breathing is loud enough that at least one of your immediate theater- or concert-going neighbors would want to hush you.

• Try this breathing technique on your next walk. (It may be used in conjunction with the practice in the previous chapter.) You may be amazed at the difference you feel in your level of vitality and the ability of your mind to think clearly. If possible, use this exercise once, five to twenty-one minutes per day.

• In the event that you have difficulties mastering this technique, find a qualified yoga instructor for support. Mastering this breathing technique is fundamental to uncovering who you are.

Note: In discussing the ideas of honoring the body and the breath, there is one additional point worth addressing—that of the contracted relationship. Sometimes, we find ourselves in contracted relationships, which do not seem to be working toward the enhancement of our vitality. If you feel that an existing contracted relationship is inappropriate for you, approach someone about contract amendment, suspension or cancellation. If you are not in personal danger, ask yourself what you are learning in the given situation and conclude your contract in a timely and professional manner.

In the meantime, maintain vitality through other activities that are close to your heart, stay focused on your internal conceptual shifts and listen to your body for ideas about the best way or ways in which to proceed or redirect. Return to the twin questions: Who am I? And, why am I here? Hints and ideas will present themselves during the quiet times when you are actively attending to your body and breath.

.

Recommended Miscellany

Cooper, David A. *Three Gates to Meditation Practice: A Personal Journey Into Sufism, Buddhism and Judaism.* Skylight Paths Publishing: Woodstock, Vermont, 2000.

Cooper's introspective, autobiographical account of his spiritual journey is one of the most well written, thematic memoirs I can recommend. Cooper's book also serves as a *Who's Who* on meditation and spiritual seeking in the 1970s United States. If you want to know what having a dedicated meditation practice is like, this is one of the best and most accessible descriptions.

Desikachar, T.K.V. *The Heart of Yoga: Developing a Personal Practice.* Inner Traditions International: Rochester, Vermont, 1999.

Desikachar's honesty and thoughtfulness pervade this book on the philosophical principles behind the practice of hatha yoga. It is an excellent resource for those already immersed in their practice, as well as enthusiastic beginners.

Feild, Reshad. *The Last Barrier: A Journey into the Essence of Sufi Teachings.* Lindisfarne Books: Great Barrington, Massachusetts, 2002.

Articulate and thoughtful, this twenty-fifth-anniversary edition, with a forward by Coleman Barks (best known for his translations of Rumi's works), is an exceptional window into what it means to surrender the ego. Feild's narrative highlights the complex nature of the very classic student-teacher relationship in a non-Western setting. If you have ever encountered spiritual doubt along your path, use this sometimes exotic and urgent narrative to banish it.

Hoff, Benjamin. *The Te of Piglet.* Penguin Books: New York, New York, 1993.

The Taoist teaching tales, woven throughout the book's text, are a treasure. If for no other reason, pick up a copy at the library and read it for these intermittent delights.

Iyengar, B.K.S. *Light on Pranayama: The Yogic Art of Breathing.* Crossroad Publishing Company: New York, New York, 1994.

This book gives detailed instruction on breathing techniques in the yogic tradition. One of the most thorough works available, students and teachers of yoga alike are indebted to B.K.S. Iyengar for the gift of this book and his *Light on Yoga*, featuring yoga's physical postures.

Khan, Hazrat Inayat. *Personality: The Art of Being and Becoming.* Omega Publications: New Lebanon, New York, 1989.

In many respects Hazrat Inayat Khan is considered the father of ecumenical Sufism in the West. This book is from *The Collected Works of Hazrat Inayat Khan.* Many volumes from the original collection are available in print and others are accessible online. Originally presented early in the last century, the concepts remain current and applicable.

Pilates, Joseph. *The Universal Reformer.* [Equipment]: New York, New York, [c. 1923].

This citation features an original piece of exercise equipment designed by Joseph Pilates (1880-1967). If you have not had the opportunity to work on a piece of Pilates' equipment, find a trained instructor and enroll. The benefits gained by studying Pilates' "muscle contrology" with the aid of his equipment and a well-qualified instructor are remarkable.

Prakash, Prem. *The Yoga of Spiritual Devotion: A Modern Translation of the Narada Bhakti Sutras*. Inner Traditions International: Rochester, Vermont, 1998.

Prakash's treatment of this text is a boon for speakers of American English. The lifestyle recommendations given in the sutras mirror those supported by current lifestyle, science and theory experts. There are many references to traditional yogic works.

Shah, Idries. *The Sufis*. Random House: New York, 1971.

The Sufis contains a valuable overview of principles and insights into such things as Saint Francis of Assisi's mysterious wanderings about the Middle East in the late Middle Ages. The introduction by Robert Graves is a treasure of perspective and information. Also recommended is Shah's *Tales of the Dervishes*, which is a joyful series of universal teaching tales and less esoteric than *The Sufis*.

Taylor, Jill Bolte. *My Stroke of Insight: A Brain Scientist's Personal Journey.* Viking: New York, New York, 2006.

Among the many books available, discussing the nature and functions of our brain's individual hemispheres, this is one of the books I have enjoyed the most. The text, which is grounded in the Western medical model, is a forthright personal narrative combining hard science with accessibility. Taylor's gift for teaching lights the way through the entire piece.

Index

114

Acknowledgements

I would like to acknowledge the gracious and timely assistance extended by the many individuals who read the manuscript for errors, made editorial suggestions and practiced the featured breathing techniques: Maridel Allinder, Greg Hoffman, David Ketchum, Holly Ketchum, Charles Lawrence and Susan Robords. Also, thank you to the Springfield-Green County Library District's phenomenal reference librarians. Each of you worked with unflagging professionalism, expertise and patience toward the completion of this project—whether researching questions, assisting me with the recreation of bibliographic entries for books, which have long since passed through my library, or fulfilling requests for uncommon and out-of-print materials.

Julian Lynn, MFA, CEP, ERYT, is a student and seeker, who has read and studied in the areas of history, English, fine arts and hatha yoga. Recently, she spent five years in the American Southwest, teaching yoga, practicing pranic work and continuing to learn about life's beauty, vision and the importance of being. Ms. Lynn offers programs on conscious living and workshops in the hatha yoga tradition. Her greatest joy comes from assisting individuals, who are striving to enhance and expand their experiences of the Self. You may find her work at www.julianlynn.com.

* 9 7 8 0 5 7 8 1 2 0 9 7 3 *